Low Carb Diet

Fitness Secrets for Weight Loss and Improved Physical and Mental Health

(BONUS: 20 Low Carb Recipes for Fast & Easy Results)

I0435782

Table of Contents

Introduction

I want to thank and congratulate you for purchasing this book. This book contains proven steps and strategies to help you make use of a low-carb diet to lose weight and stay healthy.

It seems that most people nowadays are only interested in "quick fix" solutions to their fitness problems. Many have tried fad diets that claim to help them lose a ridiculous amount of weight in a matter of weeks.

I am not interested in those fad diets, and you shouldn't waste your time or money on them. This book isn't designed to be a typical fad diet book and won't claim that you'll lose 30 pounds of fat in 2 weeks.

However, if you gain an understanding of how carbs work in the body, you will make better nutritional decisions and achieve your fitness goals much faster. A person who succeeds will have approached the information in this book with the intent of making a *lifestyle change for the better*, not just going on a diet for a few weeks.

You will find that healthy eating is quite simple, but it does take discipline and commitment. It's about becoming more conscious of what you consume and how much of it you eat on a daily basis.

If you wish to embark on a new journey in fitness, you have to be willing to commit for the long haul, not just for a few weeks.

In this book, we will talk about the benefits of a maintaining a low-carb diet and why it works so well.

Thanks again for downloading this book, I hope you enjoy it!

Chapter 1: The Basics of Carbohydrates

Before we get started, we need to gain a basic understanding of what carbs are, how they work in the body, and when to eat them.

It is important to understand that our bodies need carbs to survive! Carbohydrates are our bodies' main source of energy.

The carbs that we eat are made up of long chains of glucose molecules that are all linked together by chemical bonds.

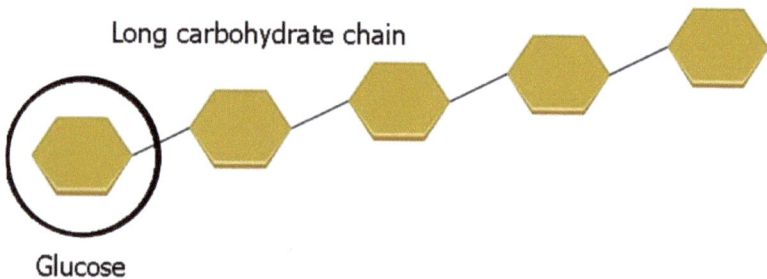

Long carbohydrate chain

Glucose

When we eat a meal containing carbs, our bodies' take the long chains and enzymatically break the chemical bonds in order to release all the individual glucose molecules. This occurs in the small intestine and is called **carbohydrate digestion**.

The glucose molecules are absorbed through the wall of the small intestine and into the blood stream. When glucose enters the blood stream it is stored in the muscles and liver as glycogen. Glycogen provides an energy source to our muscles when we exercise them.

Glycogen is broken down through a long series of biochemical pathways to make ATP.

ATP is an extremely important molecule because it fuels every biochemical function of our bodies. Our muscles need ATP in order to contract. Without it, we wouldn't be able to move at all!

This is one of the reasons why our bodies need carbs to survive.

Now, the problem with most foods today is that they are processed and contain WAY too much glucose. When we eat too much glucose, our bodies fill up our glycogen reserves first and then store all the excess glucose as fat.

This process happens after large amounts of the hormone **insulin** are secreted by the pancreas.

Insulin is referred to as the "fat-storage hormone", and it is secreted when our blood glucose levels get too high.

In order for a person to maintain a healthy weight, his or her body must not exceed its glucose requirements. An optimal blood glucose level will help a person get to a healthy weight quickly.

While at an optimal blood glucose level, the body will use its <u>fat reserves</u> as fuel. This is the secret to healthy weight loss and the heart of the low-carb diet!

Naturally, one can assume that *consuming the right* **amount** *of carbs* is the way to go!

It is also important to note that not all carbs are the same, and one must also *consume the right **kinds** of* carbs to be successful in losing weight.

We will now discuss the major differences between the main types of carbs.

I.   STARCHY CARBS VS. FIBROUS CARBS

The first thing you need to realize about these two is that they are nearly identical. The difference between starchy carbs (starch) and fibrous carbs (fiber) resides in the types of chemical bonds that link the glucose molecules together.

The glucose molecules in starch are linked together by **alpha** bonds, while the glucose molecules in fiber are linked together by **beta** bonds.

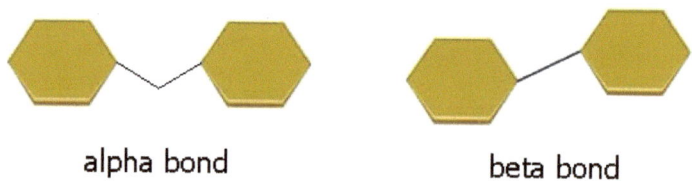

alpha bond   beta bond

Alpha bonds are weak and can be broken apart by natural enzymes in the small intestines of all mammals.

Beta bonds, however, are much stronger than alpha bonds and can only be broken down by the *microorganisms* that live in the large intestine of mammals (also in the stomachs of ruminant animals such as cows, sheep, goats, and deer).

Fibrous carbs, which are broken down in the large intestine of humans, are basically useless. This is because the wall of the large intestine lacks a mechanism to absorb glucose.

This little detail is important because eating starch will yield much more usable glucose than eating fiber will.

So, if you are trying to lose weight, then it is a good idea to fill up your stomach with fiber. You won't be as hungry, and your body won't be able to overload on glucose since it can't absorb it from fiber anyway.

This book will recommend *green vegetables* as the main source of fiber.

II. SIMPLE CARBS VS. COMPLEX CARBS

Not only can carbohydrate chains differ in bond types, they can also differ in length. Generally, carb chains of only 1 or 2 units are referred to as **simple carbs** whereas carb chains of 3 or more units are referred to as **complex carbs**.

For example, sucrose, aka. table sugar, is a simple carb. It only has 2 molecular units, 1 glucose and 1 fructose, attached by a single alpha bond.

Sucrose

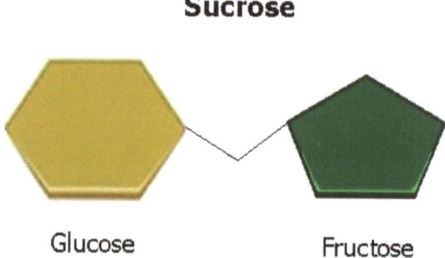

Glucose   Fructose

Starch, on the other hand, is a complex carb. It can have thousands of molecular units attached by thousands of bonds.

Complex carb

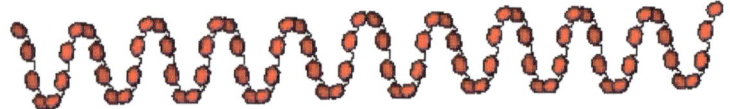

The body digests simple carbs rapidly which results in a huge spike in blood glucose levels and insulin. It takes the body a lot longer to digest complex carbs, so the elevation in blood glucose levels is spread throughout a longer period of time.

This makes complex carbs much healthier than simple carbs.

III. GLYCEMIC INDEX VALUES OF FOOD

Every type of food has a **glycemic index** value assigned to it. The glycemic index system ranks foods on a scale of 0 to 100 based on how rapidly they cause a spike in insulin.

A food type with a high glycemic index value will cause a sharp spike in insulin whereas a food with a low glycemic index value will cause a more gradual rise in insulin and blood glucose levels.

For example, black beans have a glycemic index of 30, whereas Graham crackers have a glycemic index of 74.

If a person consumes 40 grams of carbs from Graham crackers, he or she will experience a large spike in blood glucose levels and a sudden crash after an hour or so.

If the same person consumes 40 grams of carbs from black beans, he or she will experience a slight increase in glucose levels that will last for several hours with no crash.

It is important to avoid foods with high glycemic index values because they promote fat gain.

Alright, enough talk about biochemistry, let's explore the benefits of a low-carb diet.

Chapter 2: The Benefits of Limiting Carbohydrate Intake

Okay! Now that you have a basic understanding of carbs, we are going to switch gears and talk about the benefits of choosing a low-carb diet.

1. Fast Weight Loss

This is one of the primary reasons as to why people try low-carb diets. They are so effective for shedding pounds, even for people who typically struggle with weight loss.

Remember, whenever we consume foods containing sugar and carbohydrates, the hormone insulin is released. Its jobs is to signal our cells to store any available energy; first as glycogen, and then as fat.

By significantly reducing carbohydrates in our diet, as well as keeping our body's glycogen stores low, we can actually prevent insulin from getting released and eventually storing fat.

The less insulin we have circulating in our bloodstream, the more our body is forced to use up all of its glycogen stores, reaching into fat stores for ongoing fuel—hence burning all of it up.

2. Better Cognitive Function

Most people consume way too many carbs, and they prevent their bodies from absorbing healthy fatty acids. This is problematic because we all require healthy fats in order to achieve proper brain function, mood control, and optimal hormone regulation.

While a sugary or high-carb meal can certainly make you feel more alert for a period of time, this only lasts for a short while and you'll eventually come crashing down-- feeling tired, lethargic and irritable.

Healthy fats serve as antioxidants as well as precursors to a number of important brain-supporting neurotransmitters and molecules that control our learning, mood, memory and energy.

In fact, our brains are largely composed of these fatty acids, and they require a steady supply of fats from our daily diet in order to perform efficiently.

3. Reduced Risk of Metabolic Syndrome and Heart Disease

Research has proven that low-carbohydrate diets are much more effective at reducing heart disease risk factors when compared to low-fat diets.

A specific study showed that both low-carb and low-fat diets are capable of helping with weight maintenance and improving an individual's metabolic risk factors.

However, participants on low-carb diets actually experienced a greater increase in "good" high-density lipoprotein and a greater reduction in triglycerides when compared to participants on low-fat diets.

4. Lower Risk for Type-2 Diabetes

This is a particularly interesting benefit—given that diabetes affects quite a significant portion of the population.

A growing body of evidence suggests that low-carb diets are much more effective at reducing one's risk for Type-2 Diabetes than typical low-fat/high-carb diets.

Since Type-2 Diabetes is caused by resistance to insulin, low-carb diets can prevent this disease by keeping insulin levels low.

5. Fewer Cravings and Less Hunger!

Cravings are the biggest challenge that most dieters face. However, this becomes much less of a worry once they switch to a low-carb diet.

A low-carb diet actually turns off the production of "Ghrelin" also known as the "Hungry hormone." According to studies, insulin negatively impacts this hormone—leading to constant cravings.

Since carbs spike insulin levels in the body, they also trigger the production of ghrelin which will make you crave more food even after you've eaten a lot.

On the other hand, fats and proteins allow you to go for longer periods of time without needing another snack or a meal.

This is because fats and proteins do not activate ghrelin production, and they provide you with a more nutritionally-filling diet.

6. Better Digestion

Last but not the least, a diet that's low in carbs can also lead to much better digestion and prevent digestion-related problems.

This is because sugar actually feeds the bad bacteria in our digestive system—too much of which can result in a number of issues such as indigestion, leaky gut syndrome, and diarrhea.

To counteract this problem, eat plenty of quality proteins and healthy unsaturated fats.

Fat-burning foods can also nourish our digestive tract and reduce the growth of harmful bacteria.

Chapter 3: Grocery List For a Low-Carb Diet

Produce Aisle

- Salad greens such as: lettuce, spinach and cabbage. You can also include other popular leafy greens such as Swiss chard or other chard, collard greens, bok choy, and kale.

- Herbs like basil, parsley, and cilantro.

- Vegetables such as radishes, cucumbers, sprouts, and tomatoes can be used for side dishes as well as salads.

- Green vegetables such as cauliflower, avocado, okra, asparagus, Brussels sprouts, broccoli, and green beans.

- Non-starchy veggies such as eggplant, mushrooms, summer squashes, artichokes, green onions, and peppers.

- If fruit is allowed in your chosen plan, adding a few servings of berries, some melons, and even small peaches should be good.

Poultry, Meat, Seafood and Eggs

- These should all be fine for a low-carb diet; eggs are very nutritious and they can be eaten and cooked in many different ways. Liver and oysters do contain a bit of carbs, so eat them in moderation.

Dairy

- Butter, cream, full-fat cottage cheese, ricotta, sour cream, cheeses, and sugar-free yogurt.

Fats and Oils

- Butter
- Coconut oil
- Olive oil
- Sunflower and safflower oils
- Sesame and other types of nut oils
- Nut butters

Frozen Foods

- Keep frozen meats, fish, vegetables, and berries handy.

Condiments

- Mustard, sugar-free ketchup, mayo, sugar-free relish, salad dressings, broth or bouillon, soy sauce, spices, pesto sauce, hot sauce, sugar-free preserves, and jams.

Other:

- Unsweetened soy

- Rice

- Almond

- Pork rinds

- Hemp Milk

- Low-carb tortillas

- Unsweetened chocolate

- Unsweetened coconut

- Cocoa powder

On a moderate-carb diet you can add limited amounts of: corn, high-fiber breads, al dente pasta and grains such as quinoa, barley, and oats. You can also add a little more fruits.

Chapter 4: Easy Low-Carb Recipes

For the diet to work, you will have to apply a number of changes to your lifestyle—especially to the food you consume on a daily basis.

In this chapter, you will be provided with 20 simple yet filling dishes that will take your weight loss and health to a whole new level.

Shall we begin with the most important meal of the day?

Bon appétit!

BREAKFAST RECIPES

1. <u>Eggs and Veggies Fried in Coconut Oil</u>

Ingredients:

- Spinach

- Coconut Oil

- Eggs

- Frozen/Fresh Vegetable Mix

- Spices

Instructions:

- Add a moderate amount of **coconut oil** to your frying pan and turn up the heat.

- After it gets warm enough, toss in your vegetables. Add eggs and spices.

- Add spinach.

- Stir fry until ready.

2. Healthy Breakfast Skillet

Ingredients:

- 1 lb. breakfast sausage

- 2 eggs

- 2 diced sweet potatoes

- A handful of cilantro

- 1 diced avocado

- Hot sauce

- Raw cheese (optional)

- Salt and pepper

Instructions:

- Start by preheating your oven to 400°F.

- Taking an oven-safe skillet, crumble and brown the sausage over medium heat. Once browned, take it off the skillet and set aside while cooking the sweet potatoes. Reserve as much of the grease as possible.

- Add the sweet potatoes into the sausage grease and allow this to get crispy. Add the sausages again after the potatoes are done.

- Make two wells in the pan and crack each of the eggs into these.

- Take your skillet and place it in the oven. Bake this long enough for the eggs to set, which should take about 5 minutes.

- Turn the oven to broil for another minute or two and make sure to keep the yolk from cooking all the way.

- Remove your pan from the oven then add your avocado, cilantro and hot sauce.

3. Tex Mex Scramble

Ingredients:

- 5 eggs
- 1/8 cup green pepper, chopped
- 2 Tbsp. water
- 1/8 cup red onion, chopped
- 1/2 cup frozen spinach
- 2 cherry tomatoes, diced
- 5 jalapeno pepper slices, chopped
- 2 Tbsp. Pace Salsa
- 1 slice of pepper jack cheese (you can also use cheddar)

Instructions:

- Preheat your skillet over medium heat. Add oil of choice.
- Mix in the tomatoes, eggs, pepper, water, spinach, onion and jalapenos together. Transfer this to another pan and cook until eggs are to your liking.
- Just before removing the eggs, turn the heat off then add the pepper jack cheese on top. Cover this with a lid and set aside for 5 minutes.
- Top with the salsa and serve immediately.

4. <u>Cheese and Chive Waffles</u>

Ingredients:

- 1 cup raw cauliflower
- 1 cup mozzarella shredded cheese
- 1/3 cup Parmesan cheese/shredded
- 2 eggs
- 1 tsp. garlic powder
- 1/2 tsp. pepper
- 1 tsp. onion powder
- 1 Tbsp. chives
- Fresh parsley
- Sun-dried tomatoes

Instructions:

- Heat your waffle maker until it is ready then add about 1/4 cups filled with batter to the griddle. Set your timer for 4-6 minutes. When the waffle still sticks to the waffle maker after this much time has elapsed, allow the batter to cook slightly longer. Let these cool on a plate before serving.

5. <u>Mini Cheese and Broccoli Omelets</u>

Ingredients:

- 1/4 cup Sargento (shredded cheddar - reduced fat)

- Salt and fresh pepper

- 1 tsp. olive oil

- 1/4 cup good grated cheese

- 4 cups broccoli florets

- 4 large eggs

- Cooking spray

Instructions:

- Preheat your oven to 350° then steam the broccoli around 6 minutes.
  After the broccoli has been cooked, gently crumble it into much smaller pieces before adding some salt, pepper, and olive oil. Make sure you mix everything properly.

- Begin cooking the eggs as desired then toss in your florets. Plate this and top with some of the grated pecorino and sargento before serving.

LUNCH & SNACK RECIPES

1. <u>Ground Beef with Sliced Bell Peppers</u>

Ingredients:

- Ground beef
- Onions
- Spinach
- Spices
- Coconut Oil
- Bell Pepper

Instructions:

- Cut the onion into smaller pieces.
- Put some coconut oil on your pan then turn up the heat.
- Add the onions and stir for a couple of minutes.
- Add your ground beef then toss in some spices.
- Add the spinach.
- Stir fry everything until ready and serve this with the slices of bell pepper.

2. Paleo Lettuce Wrap

Ingredients:

- 3 tbsp. of your chosen fat or oil

- Handful of cilantro, chopped

- 1 lemon, juiced

- 1 lb. chicken thighs or breasts, you can also use ground chicken

- 1 tsp. sesame oil

- 4 oz. chopped mushrooms (shiitake)

- 1/2 onion, already diced

- Iceberg lettuce

- 2 pcs. green onions already chopped finely

- 3 cloves of garlic already minced

- 1 tsp. chili garlic sauce

- 1 avocado, sliced

- 1/4 cup soy sauce (wheat free and reduced sodium)

Instructions:

- Take a sauté pan and heat up some of the oil, and then chop the chicken. Make sure you chop it into very small pieces (just like ground chicken) before you start frying it.

- Add some lemon juice, sesame oil, chili sauce, green onions, soy sauce, and cilantro and mix in a bowl for serving.

- After the chicken is cooked, add this to the mixture in the bowl as well.

- Add some more oil into the pan for sautéing. Sautee the onion, mushrooms and garlic together until it turns into a golden color. Add this to the bowl and then toss the mixture to coat evenly.

- Peel your lettuce into separate "cups" and make sure you wash it. Place even amounts of the chicken mixture on the lettuce and top this with the avocado.

3. <u>Healthy Chili Cheese Dogs</u>

Ingredients:

- 3 sweet potatoes, sliced in half

- 1/2 tsp. cocoa powder

- 1 lb. ground beef

- 15 oz. of fire roasted tomatoes, chopped finely

- 2 cloves garlic, minced

- 6 hot dogs

- 2 pieces of Chipotle peppers, chopped

- 3 oz. raw sharp cheddar cheese, grated

- 1/2 a diced red onion

- 1 Tbsp. chili powder

- Salt and pepper

Instructions:

- Start by preheating your oven to 450°F. Then coat the sweet potatoes with a couple tablespoons of your chosen oil/fat. Place these on a baking sheet and roast it in the oven for about 10 minutes at most. This will give the skins a nice charred look.

- While the sweet potatoes are roasting, you can start preparing the chili.

- Begin by adding a few tablespoons of fat to your sauté pan. Allow this to heat up before adding the onions and garlic. Sauté these until they begin to soften-- which should take about 10 minutes.

- Toss in your chipotle peppers, chili powder, salt, pepper, tomatoes, and cocoa. Crumble all the beef into the pan then cook it thoroughly. Let this simmer until the chili is ready. Make sure you crumble up any small pieces to keep it even.

- Once the potatoes are roasted, remove these from the baking sheet and place the hot dogs on it. Throw the sheet back into the oven and cook it for about 7 more minutes or until the skins begin to blister.

- To serve, arrange the sweet potato skins on your plate then add the hot dogs on top. Spoon on a bit of chili and grated cheese to finish it off.

4. Shrimp and Avocado Salad

Ingredients:

- 3 Tbsp. Lime Juice
- 2 Tbsp. Olive Oil
- ½ cup cilantro, chopped
- 1/8 tsp. cracked Pepper, to taste
- Salt

Ingredients (Salad):

- Cilantro dressing
- 1 lb. of cooked shrimp
- 2 ripened avocados
- 4 cups lettuce or any baby greens of your choice

Instructions:

- Start by pouring your cilantro dressing over the shrimp. Stir to coat evenly as this also serves as your marinade. Cover this mix and refrigerate it for at least 1 hour.
- Wash and dry the lettuce. Divide it evenly among all the plates you're serving.
- Slice the avocado into smaller sized wedges. Sprinkle these over the lettuce.
- Top it with some of the marinated shrimp and leftover dressing.

5. Spicy Baked Cauliflower and Sweet Potatoes

Ingredients:

- 1 head of cauliflower
- 1 sweet potato, diced
- 1 tsp. red pepper flakes
- 2 tsp. cayenne pepper
- 1 yellow onion, diced
- 1 Tbsp. smoked paprika
- 1 tsp. dried oregano
- 4 Tbsp. fat of choice
- Salt and pepper

Instructions:

- Begin with preheating your oven to 375 degrees.
- Once hot enough, toss in all of your ingredients into a 9x13 baking dish. Mix everything well.
- Place this in the oven and let it cook for about 30-35 minutes or until sweet potatoes are tender.
- Serve warm.

DINNERS AND SOUPS

1. <u>BBQ Meatballs</u>

Ingredients:

- 1 lb. ground pork
- 1 tsp. paprika
- 1 tsp. granulated sugar substitute
- ¼ tsp. cayenne pepper
- ½ tsp. salt
- ¼ tsp. black pepper
- 1 egg
- ¼ tsp. celery salt
- ½ tsp. ground cumin
- ¼ cup almond flour
- 1 Tbsp. water

For the BBQ sauce:

- ¼ cup yellow mustard
- 2 Tbsp. apple cider vinegar
- 2 tsp. Frank's Hot Sauce
- 3 Tbsp. granulated sugar substitute
- 1 Tbsp. dried onion flakes
- 2 Tbsp. low sugar ketchup

- salt and pepper to taste

Instructions:

For the sauce:

- Mix all of the ingredients in a small saucepan, stirring it continuously until it blends smoothly. Allow to simmer on low heat for at least 8 minutes.

For the meatballs:

- Take all of your ingredients and mix everything in a medium bowl. Make sure that you mix all of it well. After, form it into 16 meatballs— more or less depending on the size you want your meatballs to be.

- Next, take a large nonstick pan and fry the meatballs over low heat, making sure that it is evenly golden on all sides. It should take about 3 to 4 minutes.

- Toss this lightly in the sauce then spread on a baking sheet lined with parchment. Broil this for another couple of minutes before serving. Allow to cool for a bit before serving.

2. Asian Style Chicken Wings

Ingredients:

- 3 lbs. Chicken Wings, separated
- 1 Tbsp. Fresh Ginger (chopped)
- 2 Tbsp. Extra Virgin Coconut Oil
- 1 tsp. Fennel Seed
- 4 cloves Fresh Garlic , chopped
- 1 tsp. Anise Seed
- 2 Tbsp. Sesame Oil
- ½ cup Coconut Aminos
- 2 Tbsp. Coconut Vinegar
- 2 Tbsp. Honey
- 1 Tbsp. Fish Sauce

Instructions:

- Heat coconut oil over medium-high heat then add garlic, ginger, anise and the fennel seeds. Keep stirring as you cook this so that it doesn't end up burning. Cook until fragrant which takes about 2-3 minutes.

- To it, add your coconut aminos, vinegar, honey, and fish sauce. Bring the mixture to a boil and let it simmer for 1 minute.

- Remove your pan from the heat and drizzle on some sesame oil.

- Pour this mix over the chicken wings, making sure that everything is evenly coated. Once these chicken wings have cooled enough to touch, cover it with plastic wrap then place it in the fridge to marinade overnight. During this time, stir the wings every few hours or so.

- The following day, drain the excess marinade and barbecue the wings until they are cooked as desired. You can also opt to bake these at 375 for 45 minutes to an hour, making the meat very tender and the skin really crispy.

3. ## Catfish in Butter Cream

Ingredients:

- 2 catfish fillets
- 1 shallot, finely chopped
- 1 Tbsp. olive oil
- 3 Tbsp. butter
- Juice from 1 lemon
- 1/2 cup coconut milk
- Finely chopped chives for garnish

Instructions:

- Pat your fish dry with some paper before lightly salting it. Next, heat up some olive oil over medium heat and sauté the shallots for about 30 seconds.

- Add your butter and after it melts completely, toss in the catfish. Fry this for about 4 minutes on each side—if the fish still sticks to the pan, this means that it isn't ready to be flipped yet.

- Remove it from the skillet after and turn the heat down before adding some lemon juice. Scrape up any crispy bits from the pan and add some coconut milk; let this boil for about 3 minutes, making sure that you stir it until the sauce thickens.

- Pour the sauce over the catfish and finish it off with chives on top.

4. <u>Halibut with Cilantro and Mango Salsa</u>

Ingredients:

Ginger Mango Salsa

- 1 mango, peeled and diced
- 1 tsp. fresh grated ginger
- ½ small red onion, finely chopped
- ½ red bell pepper, finely chopped
- 2 garlic cloves, minced
- 1/2 a bunch of cilantro, diced
- Juice from ½ a lime

Cilantro Sauce

- ½ cup homemade mayo
- 1 tsp. cumin
- ½ cup cilantro
- 2 tsp. lime juice
- Hot sauce

The Fish

- 2 Tbsp. of coconut oil
- 1 pound halibut
- Sea salt and black pepper

Instructions:

- Take your fish and season it on both sides with salt and pepper. Next, heat the coconut oil over medium high heat.

- Once it gets hot, place your fillets carefully onto the pan and cook it for about 4 minutes for each side. This depends upon your preferences too so cook as you see fit.

- Take the fish off the heat. Allow it to cool down for a bit before topping it with the salsa and cilantro sauce.

5. Paleo Fish Sticks

Ingredients:

- 1 ½ lbs. haddock

- 6 oz. of plantain chips

- Palm of coconut oil

Instructions:

- If you own a food processor, crush the plantain chips in it until you get the consistency of bread crumbs. If not, you can crush them the old fashioned way using a zip lock and a wooden roller. It doesn't have to be really fine, just make sure that there are no big lumps.

- Next, take the crumbs and place them in a zip bag. Add some salt—if they haven't been salted yet. Take the fish fillets and coat it with the crumbs; use the bag as a shaker to evenly coat everything. It will make the work much quicker and easier.

- Next, heat up your chosen oil over medium heat. Once it gets hot enough, place the fish sticks in it and cook thoroughly. It should take less than a minute for each side to turn gold. However, if you cut them thickly, give it a couple more minutes to properly fry.

- Allow to cool for a bit before serving.

DESSERTS AND TREATS

1. <u>Peanut Butter Chocolate Cheesecake</u>

Ingredients:

- 2/3 cup extra virgin coconut oil
- 1 cup Shredded Unsweetened Coconut
- 2 cups whole Raw Almonds
- 1 Tbsp. Coconut Flour
- 1/2 cup Almond Butter
- 1/2 tsp. Salt
- 1 1/2 Tbsp. Blackstrap Molasses
- 3 oz. 80% Dark Chocolate
- 1 Tbsp. Vanilla Extract

Instructions:

- Start by melting your coconut oil in a small saucepan on the stove on low heat. You can also do this using a microwave. It depends on your preferences. After this, line a 9×9 baking pan with some wax paper.

- Pulse the almonds in the food processor until it resembles coarse sand. This can also be done by hand, thought it will take longer.

- Add the rest of your ingredients except the chocolate to the food processor or blender and mix until it forms a kind of textured paste. Think of a crumbly nutella. After, pour this into the baking pan then refrigerate until set or at least 1 hour.

- Melt some more chocolate and drizzle it over the almond coconut base and spread evenly using a spoon until everything is coated. Place this back in the refrigerator for approximately 5 minutes before cutting it up and serving.

2. <u>Sweet and Salty Fudge Bombs</u>

Ingredients:

- 1 cup whole pecans, you can also use walnuts

- 4 Tbsp. Penzeys Natural Cocoa Powder

- 1 1/3 cups pitted dates, 16 pieces should be enough

- 1 tsp. of your favorite vanilla extract

Instructions:

- Place nuts, vanilla, dates and cocoa powder in the bowl of a food processor and mix until it begins to forms a paste. Make sure that there are big chunks of nuts and dates once you're done.

- Next, roll the mixture into small balls, roughly 1 inch each. Making sure that your hands are wet so that the mixture doesn't stick to it. Allow this to set on a baking sheet and refrigerate.

Garnish:

- Add some sea salt on a plate then carefully dip the tips of your fudge bombs into it. You can use shredded coconut on it instead.

3. <u>Valentine's Day Mousse</u>

Ingredients:

- 1/2 can coconut milk

- 4 oz. 71% cacao dark chocolate

- 1/4 tsp. vanilla or almond extract

- 3 oz. water

- Salt

- 1-2 ice cube trays worth of ice

Instructions:

- Take a medium sauce pan and place this over medium-low heat. Start breaking up the chocolate into chunks, place these in the pan and sprinkle some salt on it. Stir this with a whisk in order to hasten the melting process. Once melted, turn the heat off.

- Next, place the ice cubes in a larger bowl then add about a cup of cold water. Take a smaller bowl that fits into the bigger one, place it on top then transfer your melted chocolate onto it. Continue whisking this. Until you get a mousey consistency.

- Add some of the thickened, chilled coconut milk into the bowl, along with the extract of your choice; whisk this some more and make sure that everything is even and that the consistency is just right. Place another dollop of coconut milk on top of your mousse, then sprinkle the top with a pinch of coarse sea salt.

4. Almond Cake

Ingredients:

- 1 1/2 cups almond flour

- 3/4 cup butter, softened

- 1 cup granular Splenda

- 1/2 cup coconut flour, sifted

- 4 eggs

- 1/2 cup heavy cream

- 2 tsp. baking powder

- 1 tsp. vanilla

- 1/4 tsp. salt

Instructions:

- Place all of your ingredients in a large mixing bowl and beat everything using an electric mixer or whisk. Make sure that it gets blended evenly and that it takes on a very creamy and rich consistency. If the batter remains stiff, add a bit of water to thin it out a bit.

- Next, spread it evenly on a greased 9x13 pan and bake it at 350 for about half an hour or until it becomes golden. Check it for firmness as well; these are all indicators for knowing if the cake is ready.

- Cool this completely before serving—it is best stored in the fridge for baked goods containing almond because it has a tendency to turn moldy if left at room temperature for prolonged periods of time.

5. 3-Minute Choco Cake

Ingredients:

1/4 cup almond flour, 1 ounce

1/4 tsp. baking powder

1 Tbsp. cocoa

3 Tbsp. and 1 extra tsp. of granulated Splenda

1 tablespoon water

2 Tbsp. butter, melted

1 egg

Instructions:

- Mix your dry ingredients together in a glass measuring cup. If you're using liquid Splenda, make sure that you gradually stir it in while you stir the mixture.

- Once mixed, add the butter, egg and water—mix everything well using a whisk or a fork. Check for any lumps and make sure that everything is blended properly and that the consistency is even.

- Take a rubber spatula and scrape the batter down evenly before covering it with a plastic wrap. Cut a small slit in the center of this before placing it in the microwave for a minute, on the highest setting. It should set within this time and be cooked through, but still be moist on top.

- Allow to cool slightly before serving. You can add some whipped coconut cream on top if desired.

Conclusion

Thank you again for downloading this book!

I hope that you take the information in this book and commit to a lifestyle change of healthy eating.

The next step is to give the diet a try. See what works for you, and modify things according to your specific goals and needs. The point is to start it, and stick with it!

THINK POSITIVELY
EXERCISE DAILY
EAT HEALTHY
WORK HARD
STAY STRONG
WORRY LESS
DANCE MORE
LOVE OFTEN
BE HAPPY

Finally, if you enjoyed this book, then I'd suggest that you check out some of my other books. You can find a link to one on the next page.

I would also like to ask you for a favor!

Would you be kind enough to leave an honest review of this book on Amazon?

I would love to hear your feedback. If there was anything you didn't like about the book, please let me know, and I will make changes accordingly.

Thank you and good luck!

Preview of Drug Addiction

Chapter 2 – Psychological and Physical Costs of Drug Addiction

By definition, drug addiction pertains to the drug addict's repeated and obsessive use of prohibited drugs (or prescription drugs) and the withdrawal symptoms that manifest when access to the drugs is completely cut-off.

The costs of the drug addiction that manifest because of this compulsion are both profound and wide-ranging. Drug addiction has predominantly negative effects on both the physical and the psychological aspects of human beings. These negative effects can also trickle into the lives of people around the drug addict, like their immediate family members.

Psychological Effects

The psychological effects of addiction are attributed to the chemical changes that happen in the person's brain once he or she becomes addicted. Initially, a person may start using addictive drugs to cope with pain or stress.

Drug addiction basically facilitates a "cycle effect" wherein a person feels an extreme need to use the drug every time they encounter physical or emotional distress. This is basically what's known as **craving**.

Craving is an effect brought about by drug addiction wherein a person is extremely obsessed with procuring and utilizing the drug, with complete and utter disregard for everything else. Craving can be considered a side effect of drug addiction wherein the user is instilled with the belief that they cannot handle life or function normally without constant use of the prohibited drug.

Withdrawal from or intoxication with an illegal substance, such as amphetamine or cocaine, can bring about psychological side effects, which include suicidal thoughts or depression. Other drug addiction induced psychological effects include but are not limited to:

- Incessant desire to engage in dangerous behavior

- Confusion

- Mental Illness complications

- Violence, anxiety, extreme mood swings, paranoia, depression

Developing a tolerance to the drug and psychologically creating a need to increase the dosage

- Hallucinations

- Diminished pleasure in life

Physical Effects

Physical manifestations of drug addiction vary greatly from person to person or from drug to drug. However, these physical manifestations are clearly evident in every system of the body. The physical effects of drug addiction take place primarily in the drug addict's *brain*.

Addiction significantly alters how the brain works, which also impacts how the human body perceives *pleasure*. Most prohibited drugs incessantly bombard the brain with chemicals such as serotonin and dopamine, which cause various alterations in the brain. The brain then does what it does best; adapts and become dependent on the highs that these drugs induce.

Furthermore, the physical effects of drug addiction are not only limited to the drug addict alone. The effects can also be seen in infants of drug addicts. Babies who are born to drug-using mothers usually exhibit cognitive defects upon birth. Also, **1 in 4 post natal deaths are attributed to the effects of drug addiction.**

Illegal substances can cause various significant physical effects that range from slowed breathing and marked sleepiness, as with heroin, to the rapidly increasing heart rate induced by cocaine. Withdrawal from drugs such as PCP and crystal meth may result in seizures as well.

Other drug addiction induced physical effects include but are not limited to:

- Drastic changes in sleeping patterns, body temperature, and appetite

- Significant liver and kidney damage

- Respiratory complications such as breathing difficulties, emphysema, and lung cancer

- Contraction of hepatitis A & B, HIV, and other lethal illnesses

- Brain damage, seizure, stroke

- Diarrhea, constipation, abdominal pain, and vomiting.

- Heart attack or irregularities in the heart rate

If you or someone you are close to is afflicted with a drug addiction, then you will benefit from my book below:

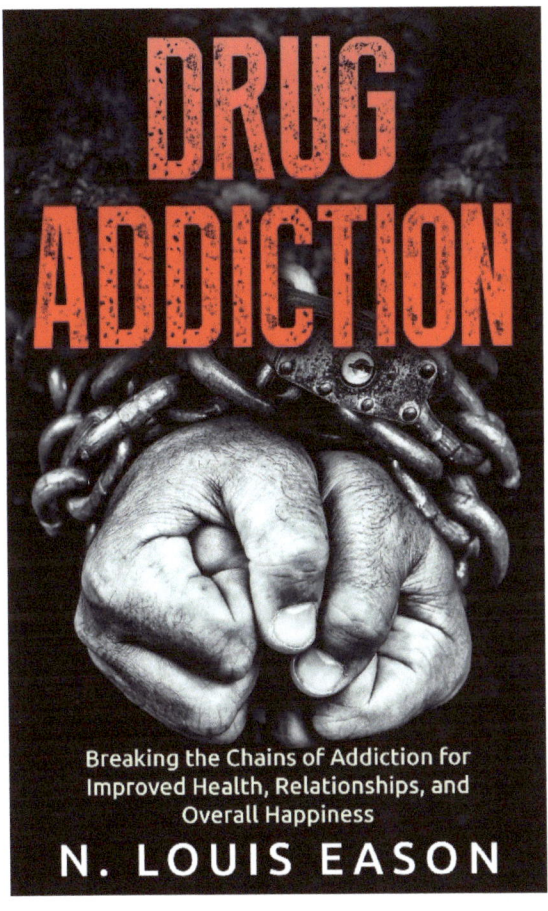

www.ingramcontent.com/pod-product-compliance
Lightning Source LLC
Chambersburg PA
CBHW040746010626
45792CB00027B/292